Dedicated
to
Health Care Professionals

Paperback ISBN: 979-8-9861693-4-7
E-book ISBN: 979-8-9861693-6-1

Exercise.

How?

(Mindful thoughts of a Personal Trainer)

Book 2

Jeff Shammah

Book's intention:

It is **not** an accident that these books (***Why*** and ***How***) are written in a philosophical way.

There are:

Plenty of excellent and well written books, with detailed exercise information available. We are overwhelmed with information **(Internet).** What is lacking are the basic skills to understand and interpret.

Books will:

Get simpler, **not** more complicated.

Will serve as:

An example of less being more.

Will promote:

Quality over Quantity.

Frequency and Severity

**are the difference between
healthy and unhealthy individuals.**

When we lack the daily practice of healthy habits in our lives we will get sick more often **(frequency)**, and the length of time and difficulty in recuperating will increase **(severity).**

When we maintain our bodies through regular exercise and healthy nutritional habits, we will experience *less* frequent and *less* severe health problems.

Not, the absence of them.

Acute and chronic illnesses can be helped (after being diagnosed and addressed by your doctor), and lead towards therapeutic exercise and hopefully recovery.

Exercise is not perfect, but it will help us to handle stress and illness better.

Where
to
begin...

Understanding the main reasons to exercise:

1. Gratefulness...

for the **gift** of life, and the maintenance of that gift (mind, body, spirit).

2. Function...

mentally, physically and emotionally, in whatever job or responsibility that life demands of us.

Secondary reasons:

- looking good
- competition, etc.

The Imagination

The unlocking and rediscovery of the imagination is key.

Are there really new and cutting edge exercises and routines?

or

Are they things that have always been there...

and have yet to be discovered?

Children

are actively developing their imaginations.

Adults

stop exploring their imaginations.

Responsibilities, stress, poverty, prejudice etc., begin to take priority...

Which in turn:

- creates barriers that are difficult to overcome.
- leading to anger and bitterness as we age.

But, because we are living longer and are exposed to technological advances, our future and our health are only limited by our **imaginations.**

Fear of aging and death often lead to poor choices in health and in life.

Since **matter** (what we are made of) does not die, but only changes form...

Then go ahead and **live**, there is nothing to fear!

Convenience:

should *not* be associated with growth.

Nothing in life worth having or retaining has ever come conveniently. Not school, not family, not career, not home, not sustained loving relationships and certainly not freedom.

Instant Gratification:

***Avoid,* when it comes to health:**

"Lose ten pounds in ten days" is *not* the answer.

Perseverance:

because exercising involves discomfort, it is one of the most basic ways to **hone (develop)** the skill of perseverance.

And perseverance is a quality needed to survive and thrive throughout life.

A healthier well maintained mind, body and spirit, will increase the chances of recovery.

Remember:

There are *no* guarantees in life, and:

"Tomorrow is promised to no one",

but the euphoria **(natural high)** that comes with being healthy and fit will enhance ***whatever*** number of years you do live.

How?

then...

What I have encountered
as a personal trainer
in my 40 years of teaching are:

preconceived notions, negative perceptions of truth,
and the inability to dream and imagine.

Therefore, all future growth and possibilities
are diminished!

My humble advice for the:

Beginner:
Youth or first time exerciser

Intermediate:
Middle aged or more experienced

Advanced:
Older age or veteran athlete.

Beginner:

Youth or first time exerciser

• Take the time and **choose carefully** who your teacher is.

• **Do not** rush through the basics of establishing core strength, proper form and alignment.

• **Refrain** from increasing your performance (weight, distance, speed etc.) too quickly.

The proper creation and strengthening of your **foundation** is *paramount* to your ability to reach your full potential.

Obviously our heart is our most important muscle (organ), but the human **structural foundation** is located in the center of the body (core).

Establishing one's recognition of the muscles that constitute the core (abdominal, lower back, and gluteal muscles), and the mental connection and use of them, is the first step.

This is easier to achieve while lying on your back, with knees bent and feet flat on the floor. Progressing to plank like postures which involve all of the core muscles, thereafter.

Refrain from starting with planks which are more difficult, and will be asking a bit too much of a novice practitioner. Who will inevitably overuse their head, neck, shoulders, arms and fingers, in an attempt to compensate for the lack of core strength.

These muscles that are over compensating, which are located around the head, neck and shoulders, are already **overworked** through **overuse** of computer, phone and technological devices.

Lying on one's back is an easier and less stressful place to start for beginners. Standing and sitting are also possible, for those who cannot lie down.

Then on to planks, once mental and physical *recognition* and *use* of the core area has been established.

There are many types to choose from. Supporting oneself on hands and knees is safer for older and weaker beginners. Then a progression to more challenging types (planks).

General exercise **will not** create a solid foundation.

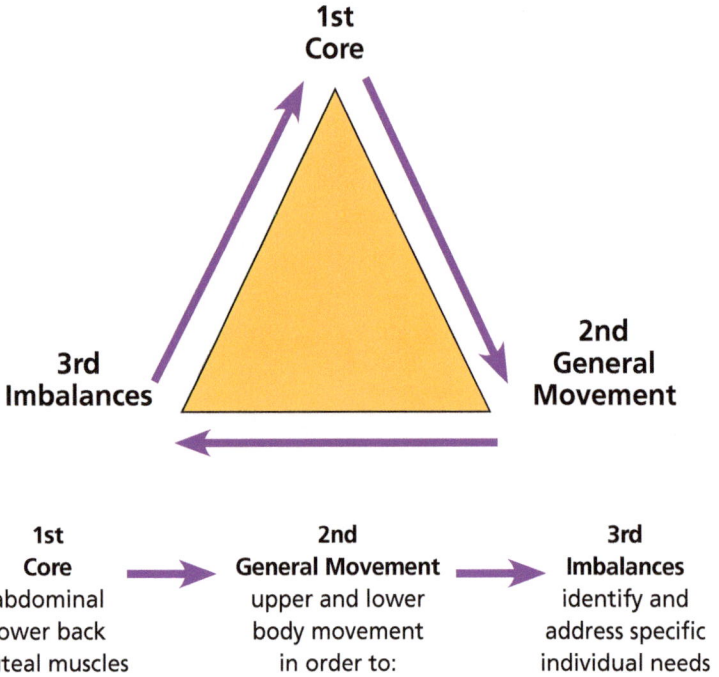

**1st
Core**

**3rd
Imbalances**

**2nd
General
Movement**

1st **Core**	2nd **General Movement**	3rd **Imbalances**
abdominal lower back gluteal muscles	upper and lower body movement in order to:	identify and address specific individual needs

Imbalances need to be identified and addressed early on, before practitioner exacerbates the imbalance through general exercise.

We need to **stop** giving out:

"One size fits all"

exercise programs, for convenience and instant gratification. Which can lead towards negative experiences and the conditioning of bad habits, that will contribute to future health problems.

Once the use of **core muscles,** basic **form, alignment** and **imbalances** have been addressed; one can safely progress through the manipulation of **intensity** (how hard), **duration** (how long), and **frequency** (how often) of any given exercise.

These principles are then expressed through the 7 Components of physical fitness:

muscular strength, muscular endurance, flexibility, balance, coordination, agility and **speed.**

All comprising a basic exercise program.

Intermediate:

Middle aged or more experienced

Change,
"The only constant in life."

We can either cooperate with change, or be dragged along kicking and screaming with it.

Either way, change will happen.

It is our choice.

For an intermediate, middle aged or more experienced practitioner, the acknowledgement of the need for change, adaptation and flexibility is necessary.

The exercises and routines in our beginner program that reinforced sound basics (core, form and alignment), will need adjusting. Due to boredom, plateaus in progress, injury and illness.

Leading to the need for Variety, which is more than just:

"The spice of life"

but, a necessary ingredient for future progress.

Since one size does not fit all, the process of trial and error as we put together our new routine, should begin again.

As I have previously stated **(Book 1)**, we should look forward to and welcome change and diversity, and the opportunity it will give us to get to know our **new** selves.

This is when our bodies begin to slow down, and we experience a gradual loss of balance, coordination, agility, speed, flexibility, strength and endurance. **Emphasizing** the need to begin the practice of training **smarter not** necessarily **harder.**

This is by no means a cop-out, or giving in to the aging process.

But an **advancement!**

Beginners need to do twice as much work, **not** because it is better, but because they lack experience.

A more experienced practitioner can begin the process of becoming more **efficient.**

The act of getting *more* done in *less* time.

This involves using prior knowledge gained as a beginner, and the knowledge of **oneself.** To form a new exercise program or routine best suited for **YOU.**

"Your exercise prescription"

This will also help in the preservation of your joints, and the lessening of the risk for overuse and repetitive movement injuries.

Transformation

Transforming

The act of reaching one's full potential, which involves transitioning from beginner (foundation) to intermediate (individual prescription), will necessitate the need for **balance** and **holisticity.**

A life long pursuit involving trial and error, which is what it means to be **alive!**

As opposed to merely existing.

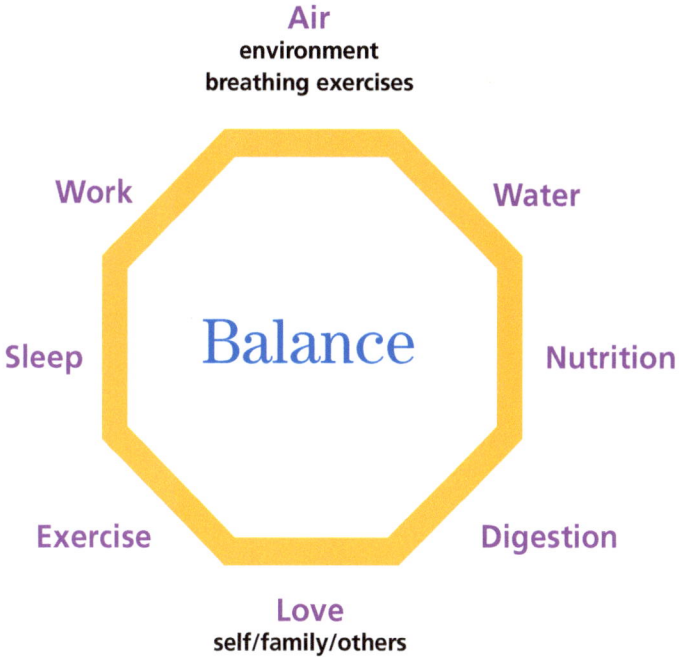

Air
**environment
breathing exercises**

Work   Water

Balance

Sleep   Nutrition

Exercise   Digestion

Love
self/family/others

Holisticity:

Improving the quality of each, with the priority placed on the area with the greatest deficiency.

Leading towards a **healthier, happier** and more **productive human being.**

Advanced:

Older age or veteran athlete.

1st
Mental & Physical
foundation
core, form, alignment
imbalances

+

2nd
Spiritual
environment
breathing exercises
meditation

The mind and body **(nervous system)** must first be exercised and balanced. Leading to a more relaxed and calm individuals ability to breathe and meditate **(stillness).**

The union of the two **(Yin/Yang)** utilizing both soft and hard exercises in equal parts, will help us achieve harmony **(balance).**

{ Gains made as we age are found by improving our weaknesses and deficiencies, **not** in a continued over reliance and overuse of our strengths. }

At this point, all that you have learned as a beginner and all that you have refined as an intermediate, begin to **coalesce** into one seamless expression of work.

Through the simplicity of exercise:

we work (move and exert force), **sweat** (release and vent), and **fatigue** (stop/stillness).

This form of discipline involving trial and error, serves as a template and foundation for all of the obstacles we will face in life.

A well rounded and progressive exercise program throughout our lives:

Mind, Body and **Spirit**

will help us live a more loving and satisfying life, as opposed to a more fearful one.

Theoretical Examples of How?

Physically Demanding High Activity Jobs

Farming, UPS, FedEx, Construction, Landscaping, Firefighter, Soldier, Police, Gardening, etc.

} *Isolated (single joint) therapeutic exercises.*

Then *general Fitness.*

High activity workers need to emphasize smaller, isolated and therapeutic exercises. That strengthen and reinforce the muscles around their joints. **Which are exhausted from the large gross** (compound) **repetitive demands of their jobs.**

• •

Less Physically Active Sedentary Jobs

Computer, Accountant, Banker, Investor, Pilot, Transit, Designer, Artist, Writer, Gamer, etc.

} *Large compound (multiple joint) movements, coupled with therapeutic exercises (carpal tunnel syndrome, etc.)*

Less physically active workers need to emphasize large gross (compound) movements. **In order to counteract the limited, isolated and sedentary lifestyle.**

Then, therapeutic exercises for their necks, backs, shoulders, elbows, wrists and fingers.

Athletes

**Professional/
Non Professional** } *Healing and Recuperation.*

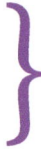

Athletes will need to change their mental, physical and emotional approach to exercise. Competition may no longer take priority. But, the **healing** and **recuperation from the overtraining and overuse injuries incurred from athletic competition,** will become necessary in order to lead a healthy and productive life.

"An Individual Health Prescription"

• •

Mother, Father, Grandparents

**Caregivers
Doctor, Nurse,Therapist,
EMS, EMT etc.** } *All of the above:
general exercise, healing and
recuperation, therapeutic exercise.*

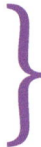

These are the **superhumans** of society. They will need to learn how to carve out time for **themselves.** In order to replenish their minds, bodies and souls, from all of the **selfless giving.**

These exercise routines will need to be **short** and **precise**,

"Time is of the essence"

Exercise modalities (options):

Calisthenics, Ballet, Dance, Free weights, Machines, Rubber bands, Gymnastics, Yoga, Martial Arts, Swimming, Running, Bicycling, Rowing, Walking, etc.

All Work!

They are not inherently better than one another.

It is the circumstance and proper use of each that matters most. Guidance from an accredited and trained professional in making these decisions is necessary and very important.

The above examples are why it is called:

Personal Training, *not* everybody training.

General Word on Nutrition

Choosing between:

Carbohydrates, Fats and Proteins

is like choosing between:

Air, Water and Food

The human body cannot function properly without *all three.*

Speak to a nutritionist to guide you on the differences between:

Carbohydrates: Simple / Complex
Fats: Saturated / Unsaturated
Proteins: Animal / Plant

It is the quality and quantity of each, not the exclusion of either.

Allergic reactions and **intolerances** to certain foods, are the reasons for restriction or elimination.

We need to stop our obsession with calories.
Caloric consumption is the fuel of the human body
(along with oxygen and water).

The elimination of them is **not** the goal, but instead the proper amount and moderation of each.

Take the time,
and get to know and speak to a:

Doctor, Nurse, Therapist, Nutritionist, Acupuncturist,
Pharmacist, Personal Trainer, etc.

{ **All uniquely qualified to guide us on this journey.** }

Hence (Book 1)

"Bring the right problem to the right person."

Gratitude

Dear Reader,

I realize that the absence of specific exercises and pictures may be frustrating for some. I wish to reiterate that I do not believe in any one "right way" to exercise. But instead, in the individual's pursuit of **self** and their own:

"Individual Health Prescription."

At some point we realize that every new exercise program or trend that seemingly has all of the answers, is actually just another piece to our puzzle. That served a purpose in our journey towards better understanding ourselves and improving our health. Unfortunately, individuals of all levels of fitness have succumbed to disease and illness. Re-emphasizing that it is the quality of our lives not just the quantity.

A healthy and properly functioning immune system, will fight on our behalf any form of injury, illness or disease that attacks our bodies.

Exercise, along with the proper consumption of **Air, Water, Food** and **Sleep**, will strengthen our immune system and its ability to prevent, heal and recover from injury, illness and disease.

So, I instead hope to encourage you to **ask questions, look for,** and **find your own way**. Through the proper use of all the exceptionally talented health practitioners out there.

Instead of just copying my way.

Choose wisely, listen, learn and be patient.

Thank you,

Jeff

To be
continued...

Credits

Photography

Susie Lang

Design

Jeffrey Shammah with Gloria Gregurovich